Contents

INTRODUCTION 4
CHAPTER ONE 5
What Is Candida? 5
   Risk Factors for Infection 6
   The Candida Diet 7
   Foods To Eat 9
   Foods To Avoid 10
   How It's Claimed to Work 12
   Getting Started — Candida Cleanse 15
   Foods to Eat 17
   Foods to Avoid 19
Sample Meal Plan 22
   Possible Benefits 25
CHAPTER TWO 27
CANDIDA DIET RECIPES 27
   Apple Cider Vinegar - Coconut Anti Candida Drink .. 27
   Anti Candida Dark Chocolate - Chia Pudding Recipe 29
   Keto, Candida-Friendly, Gut-Healing Paleo Pancakes 32
   Keto, Candida-Friendly, Gut-Healing Paleo Pancakes 36

Oat Bran-Buckwheat Carrot Cake Porridge 38

Mindful Veggie Bowl 40

Baba Ganoush (Paleo / Vegan / Low-FODMAP) 43

Nachos With Rutabaga Chips 44

Marinated Kale Salad 49

Buckwheat And Brussels Sprout Salad 51

Superfood Sesame Salmon Burgers 54

Kimchi Meatballs 56

Green Chili Chicken Stew 59

The Candida Diet Shamrock Shake 61

Candida Killing Cinnamon Cookies 64

Low Carb Chocolate Mousse Detox Recipe 67

Candida Cleanse Antifungal Energy Tea 70

Noatmeal Detox Recipe 72

Cauliflower Rice Detox Recipe 75

Detox Healthy Guacamole Recipe 78

Colon Cleanse Recipe 81

Apple Cider Vinegar Parasite Cleanse Salad Dressing
.... 84

Keto Cinnamon Waffles with Coconut Glaze 86

Keto Turkey and Egg Breakfast Skillet 90

Keto Breakfast Burger with Avocado Buns 92

"Cheesy" Broccoli Breakfast Muffins 95

Gut-Healing Garlic Asparagus Broccoli Soup 97

Light Pasta Primavera with Veggie Noodles 100

Mediterranean-Style Stuffed Spaghetti Squash 102

Slow Cooker Keto Pulled Pork Chili 105

Spinach Artichoke Grilled Cauliflower Sandwiches 108

Spicy Chicken Fritters with Creamy Guacamole 112

Baked Salmon Croquettes 115

Paleo Kale Chips 117

Easy Beet Chips 119

Crispy Golden Eggplant Fries Recipe 121

Cajun Oven-Baked Pickles 124

Easy Cauliflower Tater Tots 126

Guacamole Deviled Eggs 128

Keto Breakfast Burrito with Bacon and Avocado ... 130

Easy Baked Coconut-Crusted Salmon 133

Low Carb Bacon-Fried Cabbage 135

CONCLUSION 138

INTRODUCTION

Many types of fungi live in and on the human body, including the genus of yeasts known as Candida. Candida is typically found in small amounts in the mouth and intestines and on the skin.

At normal levels, the fungus is not problematic. However, when Candida begins to grow uncontrollably, it can cause an infection known as candidiasis. In fact, Candida is the most common cause of fungal infections in humans. Typically, the healthy bacteria in your body keep Candida levels under control. However, if healthy bacteria levels are disrupted or the immune system is compromised, Candida can begin to overproduce. The candida diet is a strict diet meant to alleviate the symptoms of candida infections.

CHAPTER ONE
What Is Candida?

Candida is the most common fungus in the human body. It's often found in areas like the mouth, skin, digestive tract, toenails, rectum and vagina. It's generally harmless, but an overgrowth of this fungus can lead to infection.

There are more than 150 known candida species living in various parts of your body. These species aid digestion and nutrient absorption from food.

Possible symptoms of an infection include:

• Nausea

• Bloating, constipation or diarrhea

• Chronic fatigue

• Skin issues such as eczema or rashes

• Recurrent urinary tract infections

- Irritability and mood swings

- Anxiety or depression

- Joint pain

Despite the large number of candida species in your body, only 15 can cause an infection. Candida albicans is the most common infection culprit, accounting for over half of all cases.

Risk Factors for Infection

There are several risk factors for candida infection, including:

- A diet high in refined carbs and sugar

- High alcohol consumption

- Elevated stress levels

- Imbalance in your microbiota

- Improper use of catheters

- Birth control pills or antibiotics

- A diabetes mellitus diagnosis

- A weak immune system

If you have any of these risk factors, try addressing them through a change in diet or lifestyle. Consider incorporating meditation or stress management into your schedule.

The Candida Diet

The Candida diet is designed to improve gut health, reduce inflammation, and boost immunity. The principles of the diet include removing added sugars, consuming fermented foods, and avoiding pro-inflammatory triggers like gluten and processed foods.

The foods to eat on the Candida diet include non-starchy vegetables, fermented foods like yogurt and sauerkraut, low-sugar fruits like blueberries, proteins like chicken and fish, and pseudo grains like quinoa. The diet is designed to provide optimal nutrition while reducing inflammation and depriving Candida albicans of the foods that it needs.

The most important of these is to avoid added sugars. People's diets these days are full of added sugars like dextrose, fruit juice concentrate, and high fructose corn syrup.

In fact, there are so many different names for sugar that we often don't even realize what we're eating.

Candida albicans uses sugar for cellular growth, to transition into its fungal form, and to create the biofilms that it uses to hide from your immune system.

Where possible, you should also avoid inflammatory foods like processed foods, alcohol and caffeine as much as possible while on your anti-Candida diet. By doing this, you can boost your gut health and speed up your recovery.

Candida overgrowth is often associated with gut inflammation, intestinal permeability (leaky gut), and chronic digestive problems. These symptoms can be addressed by a diet that is high in fiber, low in sugar, and full of anti-inflammatory foods.

Foods To Eat

The list of foods to eat includes a wide variety of healthy, nutritious food. These foods are all low in sugar, gluten-free, and unlikely to cause inflammation in your gut. The full list of foods to eat on the Candida diet includes non-starchy vegetables, low-sugar fruits, non-glutenous grains, healthy proteins, some dairy products, nuts and seeds, fermented foods, plus lots of herbs, spices, fats and oils.

You'll be amazed at the number of simple, tasty meals that you can prepare. Just take a look at our recipes section for lots of delicious ideas!

Remember to make sure that your meals are balanced. A good example might be an egg salad with a simple dressing of olive oil, lemon, and salt. This nutritious meal contains protein from the eggs, healthy fats from the olive oil, and carbohydrates from some avocado and other vegetables.

Foods To Avoid

The Candida diet foods to avoid list includes added sugars, glutenous grains, high-sugar fruits, processed foods, some dairy products, most condiments, alcoholic drinks, and refined oils.

Caffeinated drinks should also be minimized as they can worsen gut inflammation. Good alternatives are decaffeinated coffee, green tea, and chicory coffee.

There are three simple principles that cover most of the foods to avoid. If you're unsure about a particular food, just apply these rules.

Firstly, stay away from foods that are high in sugar. The most important foods to avoid are sugars and added sugars, whether they're added to your cereal or the natural sugars in a fig. These sugars can feed a Candida overgrowth, lead to chronic inflammation, and weaken your gut.

Secondly, avoid foods that contain gluten. More and more evidence is now showing that gluten causes gut inflammation, even in those who are not Celiac. Gluten can worsen the symptoms of Candida and leave your gut more vulnerable to a Candida overgrowth.

Thirdly, steer clear of inflammatory foods. A gut imbalance like Candida causes plenty of inflammation already. You don't want your diet to make it worse.

How It's Claimed to Work

Though many studies have examined the risk factors for candida overgrowth, treatment plans are inconsistent and insufficiently studied. The candida diet is claimed to be a possible treatment option.

This diet excludes sugar, gluten, alcohol, certain dairy products and harmful additives while encouraging low-sugar fruits, non-starchy vegetables and gluten-free foods.

However, most of these dietary restrictions are not supported by scientific evidence, as explained below:

- The diet excludes gluten because of claims it may damage your intestinal lining. However, there is no evidence that gluten causes intestinal damage in people who do not have gluten intolerance (celiac disease).

- Very high sugar intake may worsen candida infections in people with weakened immune systems. A high-carb diet may increase candida counts in some people, but evidence that it increases infection risk is lacking.

- The diet also excludes some dairy products. In theory, lactose (milk sugar) may stimulate candida growth by increasing acidity in your mouth, but this hasn't been confirmed so far.

- Foods with artificial ingredients, high mold content, preservatives and pesticides are also excluded. However, no evidence has linked mold, preservatives or pesticides to an increased risk of candida infections.

Alcohol and caffeine are discouraged in order to support healthy lifestyle practices and prevent dietary cheating.

Overall, this diet is designed to reduce inflammation and incorporate wholesome foods that may benefit your gut and reduce the risk of candida over time.

Still, to date, no studies have confirmed the diet's effectiveness.

Getting Started — Candida Cleanse

Before beginning the candida diet, advocates recommend going on a candida cleanse. This is a short-term diet that proponents believe will alleviate stress on your digestive tract and release toxins from your body.

While no studies support the benefits of a candida cleanse, it might help get you into the mindset for the candida diet. So far, no human studies have proven the effectiveness or benefits of detox diets or cleanses.

There are many ways to do a cleanse, but two common ways are:

• Drinking only fluids, such as lemon water or bone broth.

- Eating mainly vegetables, such as salads and steamed vegetables, alongside a small amount of protein throughout the day.

Some people may experience negative symptoms while starting a cleanse, such as fatigue, headaches, mood swings or changes in sleep patterns.

Keep in mind that the candida cleanse should not last more than a few days.

After you complete the cleanse, you can start following the candida diet's food guidelines.

There is no specific timetable for the candida diet. The diet's proponents claim that people may experience relief in a matter of weeks, while others may require many months to see a positive effect.

It's best to work with a healthcare provider when undertaking the candida diet to ensure adequate nutrient intake.

Before starting the candida diet, there are several things to consider:

• Start out slow: Instead of removing sugar, caffeine and gluten from your diet all at once, focus on removing one thing at a time to ease the process.

• It's meant to be short-term: This diet is meant to be used short-term until your symptoms have improved. It's not meant to replace a long-term diet plan.

Foods to Eat

Focus on incorporating these foods while on the candida diet:

• Low-sugar fruits: Lemon, limes, berries (may be eaten in small amounts).

• Non-starchy vegetables: Asparagus, Brussels sprouts, cabbage, broccoli, kale, celery, cucumber, eggplant, onion, spinach, zucchini, tomatoes and rutabaga (best if eaten raw or steamed).

• Gluten-free grains: Millet, quinoa, oat bran and buckwheat.

• High-quality protein: Chicken, eggs, salmon, turkey and sardines (organic, pasture-raised and wild-caught varieties are best).

• Healthy fats: Avocado, olives, unrefined coconut oil, flax oil, extra-virgin olive oil and sesame oil.

• Certain dairy products: Butter, ghee, organic kefir or plain yogurt.

• Nuts and seeds low in mold: Almonds, sunflower seeds, coconut or flaxseed.

• Herbs and spices: Black pepper, salt, cinnamon, dill, garlic, ginger, oregano, rosemary, paprika, turmeric and thyme.

• Condiments: Apple cider vinegar, coconut aminos and sauerkraut.

• No-sugar sweeteners: Stevia, erythritol and xylitol.

• Non-caffeinated beverages: Herbal teas, chicory coffee, filtered water, homemade almond milk, coconut milk (look for one without additives) and water infused with lemon or lime.

In addition, probiotic supplements may help alleviate inflammation, kill off harmful organisms and reduce the prevalence of candida and infection symptoms.

Foods to Avoid

The candida diet is a strict diet that eliminates sugar, gluten, alcohol and some dairy products. Candida diet proponents believe these foods promote candida overgrowth.

Avoiding these foods has not been proven to be effective against candida infections. However, studies suggest excessive sugar intake may worsen infections in mice with a weakened immune system.

The list of foods to avoid on the candida diet include:

• High-sugar fruits: Bananas, dates, raisins, grapes and mango.

• Grains that contain gluten: Wheat, rye, barley and spelt.

• Certain meats: Deli meats and farm-raised fish.

• Refined oils and fats: Canola oil, soybean oil, sunflower oil or margarine.

• Condiments: Ketchup, soy sauce, white vinegar, BBQ sauce, horseradish or mayonnaise.

• Certain dairy products: Cheese, milk and cream.

- Sugar and artificial sweeteners: Aspartame, agave, cane sugar, corn syrup, honey, maple syrup, molasses and table sugar.

- Nuts and seeds higher in mold: Peanuts, cashews, pecans and pistachios.

- Caffeine, alcohol and sugary beverages: Caffeinated teas, coffee, energy drinks, soda, fruit juice, beer, wine or spirits.

- Additives: Nitrates or sulfates.

Sample Meal Plan

This sample menu provides foods that are acceptable on the candida diet. Adjust this menu based on your own preferences.

Monday

- Breakfast: Scrambled eggs with tomatoes and avocado on the side

- Lunch: Turkey atop a salad of greens, avocado slices, cabbage, broccoli and an olive oil dressing

- Dinner: Stir-fry of quinoa, chicken breast, steamed vegetables and coconut aminos

Tuesday

- Breakfast: Yogurt parfait made with plain yogurt, 1/4 cup (25 grams) of berries, cinnamon and almonds

- Lunch: Thai red curry chicken

- Dinner: Salmon cakes served with steamed broccoli and a cup of bone broth

Wednesday

- Breakfast: Turkey-and-sage breakfast sausages (like these) with a side of Brussels sprouts

- Lunch: Lemon-roasted chicken served over salad greens

- Dinner: Hamburger patty (no bun), topped with avocado and served with steamed vegetables and sauerkraut

Thursday

- Breakfast: Vegetable omelet made with eggs, shallots, spinach and tomatoes

- Lunch: Leftover turkey-and-sage breakfast sausages with a side of sautéed cabbage

- Dinner: Coconut curry chicken over quinoa and steamed vegetables

Friday

- Breakfast: Omelet made with red peppers, onions, kale and fried eggs

- Lunch: Turkey meatballs with a kale salad and millet topped with ghee

- Dinner: Wild-caught salmon seasoned with lemon and dill, plus a side of asparagus

Saturday

- Breakfast: Buckwheat breakfast muffins with chicory coffee

- Lunch: Leftover coconut curry chicken over quinoa and steamed vegetables

- Dinner: Zucchini noodles topped with chicken, raw garlic, pesto and olive oil

Sunday

- Breakfast: Smoothie made from plain kefir, a handful of berries, almond butter, coconut and cinnamon

- Lunch: Chef salad of hard boiled eggs, turkey, tomatoes, cucumbers, olives and an olive-oil-based dressing

- Dinner: Chicken fajita bowl made with chicken, peppers, onions, cilantro, avocado and salad greens

Possible Benefits

Despite the lack of evidence supporting the candida diet's effectiveness, it has many potential benefits due to its focus on healthy foods.

The diet consists of whole foods that can also be beneficial for weight loss, heart health, gut function and reduced inflammation in your body. The diet also focuses on removing sugary foods, which have been linked to obesity, diabetes, heart disease and metabolic syndrome.

A diet such as this can be beneficial for anyone — even those without candida overgrowth.

CHAPTER TWO

CANDIDA DIET RECIPES

Apple Cider Vinegar - Coconut Anti Candida Drink

Prep Time: 2 minutes

Servings: 1

Calories: 120kcal

Ingredients

- 1 liter distilled or spring water (33 ounces)
- ½ lemon
- 1 tbsp raw unfiltered apple cider vinegar (15 ml)
- 1 tbsp raw extra virgin coconut oil (15 ml)

- xylitol, stevia or monk fruit to taste optional

- alcohol free vanilla extract to taste optional

Instructions

1. Squeeze the juice of 1/2 organic lemon.

2. Add to 1 liter of distilled or spring water.

3. Shake the bottle of the apple cider vinegar until the cloudy part ("the mother") is well mixed.

4. Add 1 tablespoon of organic raw unpasteurized apple cider vinegar. If this is the first time you make this drink, start with 1 teaspoon.

5. Add 1 tablespoon of coconut oil. If this is the first time you make this drink, start with 1 teaspoon.

6. Add a few drops of vanilla extract, xylitol, stevia or monk fruit to sweeten.

7. Drink first thing in the morning and up to four times a day. Always drink on an empty stomach, one hour before or after other meals or drinks.

8. Typical serving size is 1 cup (8 oz, 250 ml) each time, up to four times a day. Shake well before serving.

Nutrition

Calories: 120kcal

Anti Candida Dark Chocolate - Chia Pudding Recipe

Prep Time 5 minutes

Total Time 5 minutes

Servings 1

Calories 450kcal

Ingredients

- 1 cup pure unsweetened almond milk
- 1 oz chia seeds
- 1 oz hemp seeds
- 1 tbsp raw extra virgin coconut oil
- 1 tbsp raw organic cacao powder
- xylitol, stevia or monk fruit to taste
- ¼ tsp alcohol free vanilla extract optional
- pinch himalayan pink salt to taste optional
- ¼ tsp cinnamon optional

Instructions

1. Add 1 oz of chia seeds to 1 cup of pure almond milk. Mix well. Wait for 10 minutes. Mix again.

2. The chia - almond milk will turn into gel consistency.

3. Place the chia seeds - milk gel in a blender, with the hemp seeds, cacao powder, and coconut oil. Blend until desired consistency is reached.

4. Taste, and add xylitol, stevia or monkfruit to taste. Little goes a long way! Balance the flavor with very little himalayan pink salt.

5. To enhance flavor further, add vanilla extract, and cinnamon.

6. Refrigerate for 2-4 hours, or overnight. Enjoy!

Nutrition

Calories: 450kcal

Keto, Candida-Friendly, Gut-Healing Paleo Pancakes

The recipe for these pancakes has been LONG AWAITED, which cracks me up because they're pretty weird. Even after explaining the weirdness to you guys, I've still been getting a ton of messages to post the recipe ASAP. So, hey! Here ya go.

Since my diet is limited right now during my protocol, I'm always looking for creative ways to switch up my meals. I know a lot of people are in a similar situation. Sometimes we want a change from our usual routines, and sometimes we crave an old classic. But sometimes we feel like we can't have anything "special" because we're following a certain diet either long term or short term in order to help us ultimately feel our best from the inside out. We think we have to make sacrifices, but we don't!

I'm here to tell you that whoever you are, you, too, can have pancakes! Most likely with this super easy recipe. If not with this recipe, then there is another out there. I promise. I've taken a typically sugar-filled, time-consuming breakfast and found a way to make it quick, easy, and healthy, using hardly any ingredients at all. These pancakes are high-fat, low-carb, and oh-so-satisfying.

The reason these pancakes are kind of weird is because they're not fluffy and perfectly round, like most of us imagine our ideal stack to be. They are, however, gut-healing, full of healthy fats and protein, and ideal for balancing out your blood sugar. The exact opposite of most pancake recipes. You will not leave this meal with a sugar coma, I promise.

While I'm typically always a veggies and protein kinda gal for breakfast, there are random days when I just crave something...bread-like. Without the gluten. That's where these come in. You can either make one huge pancake (my friend did this the other day when she was testing it out), or a few smaller ones, like I did. I got 5 medium pancakes out of this recipe, so you can adjust accordingly.

With these pancakes, it's all in the toppings. The pancake itself isn't extremely flavorful, so use the toppings to give it that something'. Use these pancakes as a nice base, and then dress them up however you want! If you want, you could add some traditional maple syrup and berries. Instead, I drizzled melted coconut butter and almond butter on top, which I would highly recommend. Then I topped it off with my Cinnamon Spiced Roasted nuts, and later added a little bit of shredded coconut as well! So delicious.

Here are some ideas for toppings: shredded coconut, cacao nibs, almonds, pecans, walnuts, any other nuts, hemp seeds, coconut butter, almond butter, cashew butter, any other nut butter, blueberries, raspberries, strawberries, any other berries, jam, bee pollen... be creative!

As mentioned, I love these because they're compliant with so many gut-healing diets. For example, I can eat these while I'm on my protocol. They're Candida-diet friendly, low FODMAP, paleo, gluten-free, dairy-free, soy-free, and nut-free (unless you add nuts on the top). They've got a nice bit of fiber in them from the flaxseeds to make up for the lack of veggies. Eggs and flax provide healthy fats, and eggs and the collagen give you a nice source of protein to start your day!

And oh, yeah, of course I had to add collagen in there! I'm always looking for sneaky ways to get collagen into my meals. Vital Proteins is my favorite. I used the Vanilla Collagen, which gives a delicious vanilla coconut flavor to these panners, but you can also use the plain collagen and add vanilla, or just use the plain alone. You can also sub with protein powder! My one friend literally used glutamine instead... Talk about gut-healing pancakes!

Keto, Candida-Friendly, Gut-Healing Paleo Pancakes

Serves: 1

Time: Under 10 minutes

Ingredients:

- 2 large eggs

- 1.5 tbsp ground flaxseeds

- 1 scoop Vital Proteins Vanilla Collagen (or sub Vital Proteins regular collagen plus 2 tbsp vanilla, or sub protein powder of choice)

- dash of cinnamon

- dash of pink salt

- some coconut oil for your skillet

- Toppings: any you want! Nut butter, berries, nuts, shredded coconut, cacao nibs, etc.

Instructions:

1. Mix the eggs, flax, collagen, cinnamon, and salt together in a bowl and let sit for 5 minutes to thicken a bit. (If you want to be fancy, I recommend mixing some toppings into the batter! Cacao nibs, shredded coconut, even berries…)

2. Heat up the coconut oil in your skillet until melted and covering the skillet. Pour the batter into the skillet in circles to make the pancakes however large you want.

3. Let the pancakes cook until the edges are cooked and the bottom is slightly browned. Flip and repeat

until the other side is cooked. Continue until you've used all the batter.

4. Add your toppings and enjoy!

Oat Bran-Buckwheat Carrot Cake Porridge

INGREDIENTS

- 40g oat bran

- 40g roasted buckwheat porridge flakes

- 400g water

- 50g soy milk

- 1 tsp. (not heaped) cinnamon

- ½ tsp. (not heaped) ginger powder

- ¼ tsp. gingerbread spice or cardamom (optional)

- Himalayan salt to taste

- Sweetener of choice to taste (brich xylitol or stevia)

- 50g of finely grated carrot

INSTRUCTIONS

1. Measure your oat bran and buckwheat flakes.

2. Bring water to boil.

3. Reduce the heat and pour in oat bran whisking vigorously. Keep on whisking and simmering for 6 minutes.

4. Add soy milk and bring to boil again.

5. Mix in buckwheat flakes and simmer for 1 minute whisking at the same time.

6. Turn off the heat, cover with lid and let sit for 2 minutes.

7. Add salt, taste and adjust until it is to your satisfaction. Repeat the same with sweetener.

8. Throw in cinnamon, ginger powder and gingerbread spice and mix well. Taste and adjust if necessary.

9. Finally mix in finely grated carrots.

Mindful Veggie Bowl

Servings: 2 servings

Calories: 170 kcal

Ingredients

INGREDIENTS FOR VEGGIE BOWL

- 4 cups fresh vegetables, such as cauliflower, broccoli, celery, zucchini

- 1 clove garlic, thinly sliced

- 1 Tbsp. oil, such as olive or coconut

- 1 tsp. Seasoning Mix (see below)

- 1 leaf Swiss chard, sliced into ribbons

- 2 Tbsp. sliced almonds

- Olive or coconut oil

- Coconut aminos or lemon juice

- Red pepper flakes to taste

INGREDIENTS FOR SEASONING MIX

- 1 tsp. salt

- ½ tsp. turmeric

- ¼ tsp. cayenne

- 1/8 tsp. curry powder

Instructions

DIRECTIONS FOR VEGGIE BOWL

1. Preheat oven to 400 degrees F (205 degrees C).

2. Place vegetables directly on a rimmed baking sheet, drizzle with oil and sprinkle with Seasoning Mix. Roast 10 to 15 minutes, until vegetables begin to brown.

3. In a large bowl, add roasted vegetables, Swiss chard ribbons and sliced almonds, toss to combine.

4. Serve in deep bowls, drizzle with a bit of oil, a dash of coconut aminos or lemon juice and a pinch of red pepper flakes.

DIRECTIONS FOR SEASONING MIX

1. Combine all ingredients in a jar, put lid on jar and shake well until mixed.

Baba Ganoush (Paleo / Vegan / Low-FODMAP)

Ingredients:

- 1 eggplant

- 1/4 cup tahini

- Juice of 1 lemon

- 1/2 tsp sea salt or pink Himalayan salt

- Optional: extra virgin olive oil for topping

Instructions:

1. Turn the heat on your stovetop on medium-high. Place the whole eggplant on top of the heat. Let it grill up so that it softens up, turning the eggplant after each side is done so that the whole thing grills. I leave each side on the flames for about 5-7 minutes, turn it, and continue doing so until it's

grilled all over. The skin will look "cracked" and will be soft enough so that you can peel it off.

2. Peel about 80% of the eggplant, and leave the rest of the skin on (just a little). Place it in the food processor.

3. Add the tahini, lemon juice, and salt. Puree everything in the food processor until the mixture is smooth. I like to leave a few chunks in mine for a little bit of texture, but it should be pretty smooth. Add more tahini, salt, or lemon to taste.

4. Top with olive oil for extra flavor and longevity! Enjoy!

Nachos With Rutabaga Chips

Servings: 4 servings

Calories: 272 kcal

Ingredients

INGREDIENTS FOR RUTABAGA CHIPS

- 3 large rutabaga, peeled and sliced
- 3 Tbsp. oil, such as olive or coconut (melted)
- 1 tsp. salt

INGREDIENTS FOR SEASONED NACHO MEAT

- ½ Tbsp. oil, such as olive or coconut
- 1 pound ground meat, such as beef, bison or turkey
- 1 Tbsp. chili powder
- 2 tsps. onion powder
- 1 tsp. ground cumin
- 1 tsp. garlic powder

- 1 tsp. paprika

- 1 tsp. dried oregano

- 1 tsp. salt

- 1 cup water

INGREDIENTS FOR NACHOS

- Rutabaga chips (see above)

- Seasoned nacho meat (see above)

- Red pepper, seeded and diced

- Red onion, thinly sliced

- Green onion, thinly sliced

- Fresh cilantro, minced

- Guacamole

- Plain yogurt

Instructions

INSTRUCTIONS FOR RUTABAGA CHIPS

1. Preheat oven to 400 degrees F (205 degrees C).

2. Peel rutabagas, then with a sharp knife or mandoline, slice thinly. In a large mixing bowl, add rutabaga slices and oil, toss to coat evenly.

3. Spread slices in a single layer on a lightly oiled baking sheet, sprinkle with salt. Bake 25 to 30 minutes, flipping halfway to ensure even browning. Repeat with remaining rutabaga slices.

4. Transfer rutabaga chips to paper toweling to absorb excess oil. Chips will continue to crisp as they cool.

INSTRUCTIONS FOR SEASONED NACHO MEAT

1. In a large skillet, heat oil over medium heat.

2. Add ground meat and cook until browned, about 5 minutes, stirring occasionally to break up meat.

3. Add chili powder, onion powder, ground cumin, garlic powder, paprika, dried oregano and salt, stir to combine.

4. Add water, bring to a simmer and cook, uncovered, until liquid has evaporated, 15 to 20 minutes. Remove meat from heat.

FINISHING THE NACHOS

1. Place a layer of rutabaga chips on a plate. Spoon on seasoned meat mixture, top with guacamole and plain yogurt, then garnish with diced red pepper, sliced red and green onion and fresh minced cilantro.

Marinated Kale Salad

Course: Main Course, Salad, Side Dish

Servings 2

Ingredients

- 1 large bunch of organic Lacinato kale about 4 cups

- Zest and juice of one lemon

- 1/3 cup sun-dried tomatoes in oil

- 2 Tablespoons olive oil

- 1 Tablespoon apple cider vinegar

- 1/2 teaspoon sea salt

- 1/4 cup pumpkin or sunflower seeds

- 1/2 avocado diced

Instructions

1. Wash and dry kale leaves. Remove the stems by holding the end of the stem with one hand and pulling the leaf off towards the top end with the other hand. Set the stems aside for use at another time. Chop kale leaves into bite-size pieces and place in large bowl. Zest lemon over leaves and pour in the sun-dried tomatoes (allowing a little oil from the sun-dried tomato jar to go in as well).

2. In a separate, smaller bowl, whisk together olive oil, lemon juice, apple cider vinegar, and sea salt. Pour mixture over kale.* Using your hands, massage the mixture into the leaves for about 2-3 minutes. You will see and feel the kale getting softer in your hands.

3. Finally, add the pumpkin or sunflower seeds and diced avocado on top.

4. Taste for seasoning.

Recipe Notes

If you are wary of overdressing, try pouring half of the mixture in at first, then adding more as needed. There should be enough liquid to dress all the kale leaves, but not so much that it pools in the bottom of the bowl.

Buckwheat And Brussels Sprout Salad

Servings: 4 servings

Calories: 235 kcal

Ingredients

- 2 cups water

- 1 cup whole buckwheat groats

- Pinch of salt

- 2 Tbsp. oil, such as extra virgin olive or coconut

- ¼ cup shallots, thinly sliced

- ¼ cup celery, thinly sliced

- 1 clove garlic, minced

- 8 Brussels sprouts, cut in half lengthwise

- 1 Tbsp. fresh thyme leaves (or 1 teaspoon dried thyme)

- 1 cup vegetable broth or water

- Salt and pepper to taste

- 2 to 3 leaves Swiss chard, cut across into ribbons

- Fresh herbs, such as thyme or parsley, minced

- Crushed, toasted nuts, such as hazelnuts, pecans or walnuts

Instructions

1. In a medium saucepan, bring water and salt to a boil. Add whole buckwheat groats, cover and simmer for 15 to 20 minutes. Remove from heat, let rest for 5 minutes, fluff with a fork.

2. While buckwheat groats are simmering, heat oil in a large skillet over medium heat. Add shallots, celery, garlic, Brussels sprouts and saute until vegetables begin to soften and brown (about 5 minutes). Next, add fresh or dried thyme leaves, broth or water, salt and pepper to taste and simmer covered over medium low heat for about 10 minutes. Then add the Swiss chard, stirring to wilt for about 1 to 2 minutes. Lastly, add cooked buckwheat groats to the skillet, and stir to combine.

3. To serve, you can garnish with fresh minced herbs and crushed, toasted nuts. For a salad, cool it to room temperature and toss with 2 to 3

tablespoons of extra virgin olive oil and 1 tablespoon of lemon juice.

Superfood Sesame Salmon Burgers

Ingredients:

Serves: about 12burgers

o 1pound salmon, skin removed

o 1tablespoon toasted sesame oil

o 1tablespoon ume plum vinegar

o 1clove garlic, pressed

o 1teaspoon peeled and minced fresh ginger

o ¼cup chopped scallions, white and green parts

o ¼cup toasted raw sesame seeds

o 2large eggs

o 1tablespoon coconut flour

o coconut oil, for frying

Instructions

1. Rinse salmon, pat dry and cut into ¼-inch cubes

2. In a large bowl, combine salmon, oil, ume, garlic, ginger, scallions, sesame seeds, and eggs

3. Stir coconut flour into mixture

4. Use a ¼ cup measuring cup to form mixture into patties

5. Heat coconut oil in a 9 inch skillet over medium-high heat

6. Cook patties for 4 to 6 minutes per side, until golden brown

Kimchi Meatballs

These tasty Kimchi Meatballs, served with crisp slices of cucumber and radish, are a perfect Asian-inspired appetizer.

Course: Appetizer, Main Course

Cuisine: Asian, Korean

Servings: 6 servings of 4 meatballs

Calories: 194 kcal

Ingredients

Meatballs

- 1 Tbsp. olive oil

- 1 lb. ground turkey

- 2 scallions, finely minced

- 1 clove garlic, finely minced

- 1 Tbsp. fresh cilantro, finely minced
- 1 egg yolk, lightly beaten
- 1 tsp. sesame oil
- 1 tsp. ginger, freshly grated
- 1/2 tsp. salt
- 1/2 tsp. pepper
- 3 Tbsp. kimchi, minced

Sauce & Garnish

- 2 Tbsp. coconut aminos
- 2 Tbsp. sesame oil
- 0.5 cucumbers, cut into 24 slices
- 4 radishes, cut into 24 slices
- 1 Tbsp. sesame seeds

- 2 Tbsp. cilantro, finely minced

Instructions

1. Preheat oven to 400 degrees F (205 degrees C). Brush a rimmed baking sheet with a tablespoon of oil, set aside.

2. In large bowl, mix together ground turkey, finely minced scallions, garlic and fresh cilantro, lightly beaten egg yolk, sesame oil, fresh grated or powdered ginger, salt, pepper and minced kimchi. With wet hands, form meat mixture into 24 meatballs. Place meatballs on oiled baking sheet, about an inch apart and bake 20 minutes. Remove meatballs from oven, cool slightly.

3. In a small bowl, whisk together coconut aminos and sesame oil, set aside.

4. To assemble appetizer, place a radish slice on top of a cucumber slice, then top with a meatball,

repeat to make 24 appetizers. Drizzle coconut amino/sesame oil mixture over the meatballs. Garnish appetizers with sesame seeds and finely minced cilantro.

Green Chili Chicken Stew

Servings: 4 servings

Calories: 193 kcal

Ingredients

- 2 Tbsp. oil, such as olive or coconut

- ½ cup zucchini, cut lengthwise, then into 1/2 inch slices

- ½ cup yellow squash, cut lengthwise, then into 1/2 inch slices

- ½ cup coarsely chopped onion

- 2 celery stalks, thinly sliced

- 2 garlic cloves, minced

- 4 cups chicken broth

- 8 oz. cooked, shredded chicken

- ½ cup chopped green chilies (see note above)

- 1 tsp. dried oregano

- ½ tsp. salt

- ¼ tsp. pepper

- 2 Tbsp. lime juice

- Avocado slices (optional)

- Fresh cilantro (optional)

- Lime wedges (optional)

Instructions

1. In a Dutch oven, heat oil over medium heat. Add the zucchini, yellow squash, onion, celery, and garlic and cook, stirring occasionally, until beginning to soften, about 5 minutes.

2. Add chicken broth and bring to a boil. Reduce heat and add shredded chicken, green chilies, dried oregano, salt and pepper.

3. Simmer stew covered over medium low heat for 15 to 20 minutes. Stir in lime juice just before serving. Garnish bowls of stew with sliced avocado, fresh cilantro and lime wedges.

The Candida Diet Shamrock Shake

Smooth and creamy, this candida-diet safe shamrock shake is delicious without needing any high-sugar fruits or other sweeteners. It's naturally-colored, paleo, and vegan.

Servings: 1 shake

Calories: 201kcal

INGREDIENTS

- 1 large cucumber or two small ones

- 1/2 avocado or 1 small avocado

- 1 dash coconut milk you can make your own!

- 3/4 cup baby spinach

- 1 handful peppermint leaves or 4 drops peppermint essential oil or peppermint extract, to taste

- 1 handful ice optional

INSTRUCTIONS

1. Peel and cut the cucumber(s) into small chunks, and place into a blender with the rest of the ingredients.

2. Blend until smooth

3. Enjoy!

Notes

You can add protein powder or a raw egg to add some protein to the shake. (Obviously depending upon the addition, your resulting shake may no longer be vegan, paleo, or candida diet-safe. Choose a protein powder without dairy, gluten, or sugar to keep it candida diet safe.)

Candida Killing Cinnamon Cookies

Delicious sugar-free cinnamon cookies suitable for the candida diet!

Ingredients

- 3 Tablespoons Coconut Oil, softened

- 1 1/2 Tablespoons Natural Unsweetened Almond, Cashew or Sunflower Seed Butter

- 3 Tablespoons Xylitol

- 1 Large Egg if your eggs are small, please use 2 eggs

- 1/4 teaspoon Baking Soda

- 1/2 teaspoon Baking Powder

- 1/4 teaspoon Sea or Pink Salt

- 1 teaspoon Pure Vanilla Extract

- 1 teaspoon Cinnamon

- 3 Tablespoons Coconut Flour or 5-7 Tablespoons whole grain flour, like Whole Spelt Flour

Instructions

1. Pre-heat oven to 350 degrees. In a small bowl, mix together the coconut oil, nut butter and xylitol together until combined. Add the egg and mix well. Add the baking soda, baking powder, salt and vanilla. Add the cinnamon and flour and mix until combined.

2. Scoop out the dough with a small cookie scoop and roll into smooth spheres. Place on a parchment lined baking sheet. Bake for 7-9 minutes. Allow to cool on the pan for AT LEAST 3 minutes. Enjoy!

Recipe Notes

If doing the candida diet, you'll want to verify that the extracts you use have absolutely no sugars added to them! This may be a good idea in general, but it is very important when trying to kill off yeast and sugar overgrowth.

This recipe was originally written with coconut flour. If you would like to use another flour, please make sure it is a whole grain flour (gluten-free flours could work but you will need more of it called for in this recipe). The dough should look almost like a nut butter cookie dough.

These cookies are delicious for up to 2 days, however, sometimes when leftover for several hours, the cookie ingredients undergo a chemical reaction that will turn the cookies green. It's a strange reaction due to the coconut flour, baking soda and oils used. Do not be alarmed - it's not mold and the cookies are completely safe to eat!

And for some reason they won't turn green every time, it just depends on the batch.

Low Carb Chocolate Mousse Detox Recipe

Servings 1

Calories 690kcal

Ingredients

- 1 cup pure almond milk

- 1 oz chia seeds

- 1 oz hemp seeds

- 1 oz hazelnuts

- 1 tbsp raw organic cacao powder

- 1 tbsp raw coconut butter

- stevia pure monkfruit to taste

- ¼ tsp cinnamon powder optional

- ¼ tsp alcohol free vanilla extract optional

- pinch himalayan pink salt optional

Instructions

1. Add 1 oz of chia seeds to 1 cup of pure almond milk. Mix well. Wait for 10 minutes. Mix again.

2. The chia - almond milk will turn into gel consistency. You can proceed with the recipe, put in the fridge for a few hours or overnight.

3. Place the chia seeds - milk gel in a blender, with the hazelnuts, hemp seeds, cacao powder, and coconut butter. Blend until desired consistency is reached.

4. Taste, and add stevia or monkfruit to taste. Little goes a long way! Balance the flavor with very little himalayan pink salt.

5. To enhance flavor further, add vanilla extract, and cinnamon. Enjoy!

6. For added crunchiness : sprinkle a few raw cacao nibs before serving.

Nutrition

Calories: 690kcal

Candida Cleanse Antifungal Energy Tea

Servings 1

Calories 120kcal

Ingredients

- 1 cup spring water

- 1 bag organic green tea or black tea

- 1 inch ginger root

- ¼ tsp ground cinnamon

- 1 tbsp coconut oil raw, extra virgin, 15 ml

- ½ lemon

- pure stevia or monkfruit to taste

Instructions

1. Peel the ginger root and cut to thin slices.

2. Boil the ginger in water for 5 minutes together with the cinnamon.

3. Reduce the heat, cover and allow the to simmer for additional 5-10 minutes.

4. Strain the tea into your tea cup.

5. Add the green or black tea bag for 2-5 minutes.

6. Remove the tea bag. Squeeze the juice of ½ lemon, add into the tea.

7. Just before drinking: Add 1 Tablespoon (15 ml) of coconut oil. If you have never tried coconut oil before, start with 1 teaspoon first.

8. Add a few drops of stevia or pure monkfruit to taste.

Nutrition

Calories: 120kcal

Noatmeal Detox Recipe

Servings 1

Calories 670kcal

Ingredients:

- 1 oz whole flax seeds

- 1 oz hemp seeds

- 1 oz almonds

- 1 cup pure unsweetened almond milk

- 1 tbsp coconut butter

- 1 cup water

- pinch himalayan pink salt

- pinch ground black pepper optional

- ¼ tsp ground chipotle powder optional

Veggies (optional)

- ¼ bunch spinach

- 1 cup chopped broccoli

Instructions

1. Add 1 oz of flax seeds to 1 cup of water. Mix well. Wait for 10 minutes. Mix again.

2. The flax seeds- water will turn into gel consistency. Put in the fridge for a few hours or overnight.

3. Place the flax seeds - water gel in a blender, with the almonds and almond milk. Blend until desired consistency is reached.

4. Remove from blender, and place in a large saucepan, over medium heat.

5. Add one cup of chopped broccoli and spinach.

6. Cook and stir for 5 minutes. Do not boil.

7. Add a little more almond milk if you find the consistency too thick.

8. While cooking, add himalayan pink salt, black pepper, and chipotle to taste.

9. Remove from heat. Add the hemp seeds, 1 tbsp of coconut butter and mix.

10. Place in a bowl. Add more himalayan pink salt, black pepper, and chipotle if needed. Your noatmeal detox recipe is ready!

11. For added nutrients, crunchiness and flavor, add 1 oz of your favorite fresh raw nuts or seeds.

Nutrition

Calories: 670kcal

Cauliflower Rice Detox Recipe

Servings 2

Ingredients

- 1 head cauliflower
- 1 medium red onion
- 2-4 small cayenne peppers optional
- 2-4 clove garlic

- 2 medium red bell peppers

- 2 medium carrots

- 1-2 stalk scallions optional

- 2 oz hemp seeds

- 2 oz almonds unroasted, unsalted

- 2 tbsp coconut oil extra virgin raw

- himalayan pink salt to taste

- ½-1 tsp chipotle chili powder optional

- 1 tsp ground turmeric powder optional

- 1 oz unfortified nutritional yeast Not for candida diet

Instructions

1. Cut the cauliflower into florets. Remove the stem.

2. Grade the cauliflower florets to get white rice grains size. You can use a food processor or a box grater with medium size holes.

3. Using paper towels, press the grated cauliflower to remove excess moisture.

4. Chop the red onion, garlic, carrots, scallions, and peppers.

5. Heat the coconut oil in a wok or cast-iron skillet, medium-high heat.

6. Add the chopped red onions and garlic. Sauté until onions turn light brown color, about 2-3 minutes.

7. Add the grated cauliflower and mix well for 2-3 minutes.

8. Add the rest of the veggies and mix well.

9. Taste and add the chipotle chili powder, turmeric powder Mix well. Add himalayan pink salt as needed.

10. Do not overcook the cauliflower. Keep stir-frying until all liquids are absorbed and it has your desired consistency.

11. Remove from heat.

12. Right Before Serving: Add the hemp seeds, almonds, and nutritional yeast. Mix well. Enjoy! The nutritional yeast is not recommended for the first few weeks of the candida diet.

Detox Healthy Guacamole Recipe

Servings 1

Calories 1230kcal

Ingredients

- 2 medium ripe hass avocados
- 2 small jalapeño chili peppers optional
- 1 medium chopped tomato
- 1/4 cup finely chopped red onion
- 2 tbsp chopped cilantro
- 2 oz hemp seeds
- 1 oz sunflower seeds raw, unsalted unroasted
- 2 tbsp lime juice
- 1/4 tsp himalayan pink salt to taste
- 2 medium carrots
- 2 medium celery stalks

Instructions

1. Cut the avocado in half and remove the pit.

2. Using a scoop, remove the flesh of the avocados and place in a round bowl.

3. Add the lime juice.

4. Mash the avocados until you get a smooth consistency.

5. Add the spicy peppers, tomatoes, onions, hemp seeds and sunflower seeds. Mix well.

6. Taste and add salt if needed.

7. Use the carrots and celery as healthy alternatives to corn or tortilla chips and enjoy!

Nutrition

Calories: 1230kcal

Colon Cleanse Recipe

The Detox Salad Your Gut Would Love

A complete colon cleanse meal you can easily make at home, using natural healthy whole foods.

Servings 2

Calories575kcal

Ingredients

- 1 medium head raw cabbage

- 3 medium raw carrots

- 1 small raw beetroot

- 2 cloves raw garlic

- 1-2 small hot cayenne peppers optional

- 1-2 tbsp raw apple cider vinegar unpasteurized "with the mother"

- 1 small lemon

- 4 tbsp olive oil unrefined cold pressed extra virgin

- 2 oz raw hemp seeds

- Pink himalayan salt to taste

Instructions

1. Peel the beetroot.

2. Shred the cabbage, carrots and beets. Place in a large bowl.

3. Add minced garlic.

4. Cut the hot peppers into small pieces. This is optional for spicy foods lovers.

5. Squeeze the juice of 1 lemon and add to the bowl.

6. Shake the apple cider vinegar bottle to mix the cloudy part at the bottom (the mother). Add organic raw unfiltered unpasteurized apple cider vinegar.

7. Add the olive oil and mix well.

8. Add the salt to balance the flavor.

9. Add the hemp seeds and mix.

Notes

If possible, try to use as much organic & local ingredients as you can.

Nutrition

Calories: 575kcal

Apple Cider Vinegar Parasite Cleanse Salad Dressing

Servings 2

Calories 240kcal

Ingredients

- 1-2 tablespoons raw unfiltered apple cider vinegar

- 4 tablespoons olive oil unrefined cold pressed extra virgin

- 1 medium lemon

- 2 cloves raw garlic

- ¼ tsp himalayan salt to taste

- ¼ tsp ground black pepper optional

- ½ tsp mustard optional

- ¼ tsp turmeric powder optional

- stevia optional

Instructions

1. Shake the apple cider vinegar bottle to mix the cloudy part at the bottom.("The mother").

2. In a glass bottle or a mason jar, place 1-2 tablespoons of apple cider vinegar.

3. Squeeze the juice of 1 lemon and add to the bottle.

4. Add 4 tablespoons of olive oil. Shake the bottle.

5. Mince the garlic, add to the bottle and shake well.

6. To make the healthy lemon vinaigrette version, add ½ tsp of mustard.

7. Add himalayan salt and black pepper to taste. Shake well.

8. If you like turmeric, add ¼ tsp of ground turmeric and shake well. To add a little sweetness to balance the turmeric flavor, add a few drops of stevia.

9. Add to your salad. Enjoy!

Nutrition

Calories: 240kcal

Keto Cinnamon Waffles with Coconut Glaze

Serves: 4

Nutrition facts:18 grams of protein, 12 grams of carbohydrates, 37 grams of fat

These fluffy cinnamon waffles will be your new go-to whenever a carb craving strikes. They're full of healthy fat while keeping the carb count low enough to stay keto.

Tools

- Small saucepan
- Medium mixing bowl
- Small mixing bowl
- Waffle maker

Ingredients

For the Coconut Cream Topping:

- 1/2 cup coconut cream
- 1 T coconut butter

- 1/2 t vanilla extract

- 1/8 t cinnamon

- 1/8 t monk fruit powder

For the Waffles:

- 5 large eggs

- 1/3 cup unsweetened almond milk

- 1/2 t vanilla extract

- 1½ cups blanched almond flour

- 1/8 t monk fruit powder

- 2 t cinnamon

- 1/2 t baking powder

- 1/8 t sea salt

- 1 T melted ghee for greasing

Instructions

- Heat ingredients for the coconut cream topping over medium-low heat in a small saucepan until smooth and steaming, about 5 minutes. Turn the heat off and pour into a small serving dish.

- Whisk together the eggs, almond milk, and vanilla extract in a medium mixing bowl until thoroughly combined. In a separate small mixing bowl, stir together the almond flour, monk fruit powder, cinnamon, baking powder, and sea salt. Gradually whisk the dry ingredients into the wet to form a smooth batter.

- Heat the waffle maker on medium-high setting and grease with 1 teaspoon of ghee. Once heated, pour ½ cup of batter on the center of waffle maker and close the lid. Cook about 5 to 6 minutes.

- Use a rubber spatula to gently transfer each waffle to a plate and repeat with the remaining batter. Grease with more ghee as needed. Serve waffles hot, drizzled with coconut glaze.

Keto Turkey and Egg Breakfast Skillet

Serves: 2

Nutrition facts:31 grams of protein14 grams of carbohydrates20 grams of fat

Wake up to a protein-packed turkey breakfast skillet to kickstart your morning.

Tools

- Large skillet with lid

Ingredients

- 1 T extra virgin olive oil
- ½ onion, finely chopped
- ½ lb ground turkey
- 1 cup organic tomato sauce (no sugar added)
- 2 eggs
- Salt and pepper, to taste

Instructions

- Heat the olive oil in the skillet over medium heat. Add the chopped onion and sauté until soft and translucent.

- Add the ground turkey and cook until fully browned.

- Add in the tomato sauce and continue to cook for 2-3 minutes.

- Season with salt and pepper.

- Make 2 small wells in the turkey mixture and crack the eggs into each.

- Cover the skillet and cook for 5 minutes or until the egg whites are opaque.

Keto Breakfast Burger with Avocado Buns

Serves: 1 burger

Nutrition facts:84 grams of protein6 grams of carbohydrates121 grams of fat

Boost your metabolism and burn calories with this low-carb keto avocado breakfast burger.

Ingredients

1 ripe avocado

1 egg

2 bacon rashers

1 red onion slice

1 tomato slice

1 lettuce leaf

1 T Paleo mayonnaise

Sea salt, to taste

Sesame seeds, for garnish

Instructions:

Place the bacon rashers on a cold frying pan. Turn the stove on and start frying the bacon. When bacon beings to curl, flip it with a fork. Continue cooking the bacon until it is crispy.

Remove the bacon from the pan and crack the egg into the same pan, using the bacon fat to cook it. Cook until the white is set but the yolk is still runny.

Slice the avocados in half width-wise. Remove the pit and use a spoon to scoop it out of its skin.

Fill the hole where the pit used to be with Paleo mayonnaise.

Layer with lettuce, tomato, onion, bacon, and fried egg.

Season with sea salt.

Top with the second half of the avocado.

Sprinkle with sesame seeds.

The amount to half a cup.

"Cheesy" Broccoli Breakfast Muffins

Serves:

6 muffins

These warm, grain-free treats taste like broccoli cheddar soup in a muffin!

Tools

Muffin tin

Mixing bowl

Ingredients

2 t ghee, softened + extra for greasing

1 cup broccoli florets, finely chopped

2 cups almond flour

2 large pasture-raised eggs

1 cup unsweetened almond milk

2 T nutritional yeast

1 t baking powder

1/2 t sea salt

Instructions

Preheat the oven to 350°F and grease a large muffin tin with ghee.

Stir together all the ingredients in a large mixing bowl until well combined.

Spoon the mixture into the muffin tins. Bake for 30 minutes until a toothpick inserted in the center comes out clean.

Gut-Healing Garlic Asparagus Broccoli Soup

Serves: 4

Nutrition facts:6 grams of protein11 grams of carbohydrates12 grams of fat

Load up on antioxidants with this easy and comforting soup, packed with vibrant green veggies and collagen-rich bone broth.

Tools

Large stock pot

Food processor

Small mixing bowl

Ingredients

1 T olive oil

½ cup diced onion

½ lb. chopped asparagus

½ lb. chopped broccoli

4 garlic cloves, minced

6 cups bone broth

Salt and pepper to taste

¼ cup coconut cream

1 T lemon juice

2 T chopped tarragon

Instructions

In a large stockpot, warm the olive oil over medium heat. Add the onion and cook until golden, about 4 to 5 minutes.

Add the asparagus and broccoli, and cook another 3 to 4 minutes until browned. Add the garlic and cook for 1 minute until fragrant.

Add the bone broth and bring to a boil. Reduce the heat to medium-low. Cover and simmer until the vegetables are tender, about 20 to 25 minutes. Season with salt and pepper to taste.

Working in batches, carefully transfer the soup to a food processor. Purée until completely smooth.

In a small mixing bowl, whisk together the lemon juice and coconut cream.

Scoop the soup into bowls. Drizzle with lemon coconut cream and top with tarragon.

Light Pasta Primavera with Veggie Noodles

Serves: 4

Nutrition facts: 3 grams of protein, 11 grams of carbohydrates 12 grams of fat

Indulge your pasta craving with this guilt-free, veggie-packed Paleo primavera.

Tools

Large sauté pan

Ingredients

3 T ghee, divided

1 t minced garlic

1 t lemon zest

1 T lemon juice

1 t dried thyme

4 cups zucchini noodles

1 cup shaved carrots

1 cup fresh spinach

2 cups sliced asparagus

1/2 t sea salt

1/3 cup chopped basil

Instructions

Heat 1 tablespoon of ghee in a large sauté pan over medium heat, about 1 minute. Add garlic, lemon zest, lemon juice, and thyme. Sauté for 2 minutes.

Add the remaining ghee, zucchini noodles, carrots, spinach, and asparagus. Use tongs to gently toss to coat the noodles. Cover and cook for 5 to 7 minutes, until tender.

Sprinkle on the sea salt and chopped basil. Serve hot.

Mediterranean-Style Stuffed Spaghetti Squash

Serves: 2

Cook up a delicious Mediterranean-inspired meal you can eat right in the squash - no extra dishes necessary.

Tools

Baking sheet

Large skillet

Chef's knife

Ingredients

1 spaghetti squash

1 T olive oil

1 onion, chopped

1 garlic clove, minced

1 T Italian spices

1 cup mushrooms, sliced

1 zucchini, cubed

1 red pepper, cubed

2 cups tomatoes, diced

13 oz. jar of artichoke hearts, drained and sliced

½ cup black olives, sliced

¼ cup fresh parsley

Salt and pepper, to taste

Instructions

Preheat the oven to 350°F. Line a baking sheet with parchment paper.

Slice the squash in half and remove the seeds from the center of the squash. Place both halves onto the baking sheet, flesh-side down. Bake for 45 minutes or until meat is tender. Let it cool before removing the flesh with a fork, keeping the skin intact.

In a large skillet over medium heat, add olive oil and sauté onion until translucent.

Add garlic, zucchini, pepper, mushrooms, artichoke and Italian herbs. Continue cooking for five minutes.

Next, add the squash flesh, black olives, and tomatoes. Cook for another five minutes, then season with salt and pepper.

Serve in reserved squash skin and garnish with fresh parsley.

Slow Cooker Keto Pulled Pork Chili

Total time:

Serves: 8

Nutrition facts:30 grams of protein18 grams of carbohydrates11 grams of fat

Make this hearty bowl of tender, slow-cooked keto pork chili with only 10 minutes of prep.

Tools

Large mixing bowl

6-quart slow cooker

Blender

Ingredients

2 cups crushed tomatoes

½ cup coconut milk, divided

6 garlic cloves, minced

3 T smoked paprika

2 T cumin seeds

½ T chipotle powder

2 T dried minced onion

½ t salt, plus extra to taste

¼ t ground black pepper, plus extra to taste

2 lbs. pork loin roast

1 lime, divided

1 avocado

¼ cup chives

Instructions

In a large mixing bowl, whisk together the crushed tomatoes, half of the coconut milk, garlic, smoked paprika, cumin seeds, chipotle powder, salt, and pepper to taste until combined.

Pat the roast dry then season with salt and pepper. Poke the roast on all sides with the tip of a sharp knife then transfer to the slow cooker.

Top the roast with the tomato mixture. Cover and cook on low for 8 to 10 hours, until the pork is tender and cooked through.

Juice half of the lime and cut the other half into wedges. Shred the pork.

Just before serving, combine the avocado, lime juice, and the remaining coconut milk in a blender and process until smooth.

Scoop the chili into a bowl and garnish with lime wedges, avocado cream, and chives.

Spinach Artichoke Grilled Cauliflower Sandwiches

Serves: 2

Nutrition facts:33 grams of protein52 grams of carbohydrates40 grams of fat

Elevate the classic grilled cheese with this dairy-free take, loaded with artichokes and antioxidant-rich spinach.

Tools

Medium saucepan

Food processor

Medium cast iron skillet

Ingredients

1 cup raw cashews

¾ cup unsweetened almond milk

1 T nutritional yeast

1 t minced garlic

½ t salt

1 cup artichoke hearts, halved

1 T tapioca starch

2 cups spinach leaves

1 t ghee

4 slices cauliflower bread (recipe linked above)

Instructions

Bring the cashews and 2 cups of water to a boil in a medium saucepan over medium-high heat for about 7 minutes. Continue to boil for 3 minutes longer.

Drain the water and transfer the cashews to a food processor with the almond milk, nutritional yeast, garlic, and sea salt. Blend until smooth and creamy, about 1 minute. Add the artichokes and pulse 3 times to break them up slightly.

Return the cashew mixture to the saucepan and heat over medium-low heat until steaming, about 3 minutes. Gradually stir in the tapioca starch to thicken.

Once the tapioca starch is incorporated, add the spinach. Heat for 3 to 4 minutes longer to wilt the spinach. Turn the heat off and cover to keep warm.

Heat the ghee in a medium cast iron skillet over medium heat for 3 minutes. Add 2 slices of bread and toast for 3 to 4 minutes on each side. Repeat with the remaining slices of bread.

Spread 1 slice of toasted bread with ½ cup spinach artichoke mixture and place a slice of bread on top. Repeat with the other 2 slices. Serve hot

Spicy Chicken Fritters with Creamy Guacamole

Serves: 4

Nutrition facts: 29 grams of protein, 7 grams of carbohydrates, 22 grams of fat

Enjoy the flavor of tacos stuffed into hand-held chicken fritters, complete with a creamy guacamole dip.

Tools

Medium cast iron skillet

Blender / Food processor

Medium mixing bowl

Ingredients

For the Guacamole Dip:

⅔ cup mashed avocado

¼ cup Paleo mayonnaise

2 T lime juice

¼ t salt

1 T finely chopped cilantro

For the Fritters:

1 lb. ground chicken breast

½ cup almond flour

1 large egg

¼ cup chopped cilantro

2 T minced jalapeño

1 t ground cumin

1 t chili powder

¼ t garlic powder

½ t sea salt

1 T avocado oil

Instructions

Combine the avocado, mayonnaise, lime juice, and sea salt in a blender or food processor and blend until smooth and creamy, about 15 seconds. Transfer to a small bowl and stir in the cilantro. Refrigerate until ready to serve.

Combine all the ingredients for the fritters except the oil in a medium mixing bowl. Mix thoroughly.

Heat the oil over medium heat in a medium cast iron skillet for 3 minutes. Scoop 2 tablespoon mounds of chicken mixture onto the skillet, then gently flatten and shape into a circle. You should be able to cook 3 fritters at a time.

Cook for 4 to 5 minutes a side. Repeat with the remaining mixture. Serve the fritters hot with guacamole dip.

Baked Salmon Croquettes

Serves: 20 croquettes

Salmon croquettes are coated in almond meal and baked for a crispy treat that only tastes fried.

Tools

Baking sheet

Parchment paper

Mixing bowl

Ingredients

1 lb wild-caught salmon, skinless

1 1/2 cups almond meal, divided

1 egg

1 T fresh chives, minced

2 garlic cloves, minced

1 t lemon zest

1/2 t sea salt

Instructions

Preheat the oven to 400°F and line a baking sheet with parchment paper.

Lightly grease a pan with olive oil and heat over medium heat. Add salmon and cook for 5 minutes each side or until fully cooked. Shred the salmon using a fork in a mixing bowl.

Add 1 cup of the almond meal, egg, chives, garlic, lemon zest and sea salt. Form the mixture into golf ball-sized croquettes.

Roll in the remaining 1/2 cup almond meal and place on prepared sheet. Bake for 20 minutes, and serve hot with your favorite dipping sauce.

Paleo Kale Chips

Total time:20 mins

Cook Time:15 mins

Prep Time:5 mins

Serves:2-3 servings

Use this easy recipe to transform those fibrous little greens into delicate and salty crisps.

Ingredients

- 1 bunch fresh kale, curly variety
- 2-3 T extra virgin olive oil
- 1 t paprika (optional)
- Generous pinch of salt

Instructions

- Preheat your oven to 275-300 degrees F.

- While your oven is heating up, remove any large stems from the kale, and cut or tear the leaves up into littler bite-sized pieces. Remember to dry it thoroughly.

- Toss the kale, extra virgin olive oil, paprika, and salt in a salad bowl until the leaves are evenly coated and everything is nicely distributed.

- Spread the leaves out on a baking tray and cook until deliciously crispy. This will usually take 10-20 minutes depending on the strength of your oven, so keep a watchful eye on your batch to prevent overcooking.

Easy Beet Chips

Serves: 1 - 2

Nutrient-rich, colorful beets easily roast into a crispy chip. Season them lightly or heavily for an earthy snack.

Tools

  Mandolin or knife

  Baking sheet

  Mixing bowl

Ingredients

4 beets

1 tbsp olive oil

½ tsp salt

Instructions

Preheat oven to 375°F.

Using a mandolin, thinly slice beets. I set mine to 1.5 mm. You can also try thinly slicing them with a knife, but a mandolin works a bit better.

Once sliced, place in a bowl and drizzle with olive oil and salt; stir.

Line baking sheet with beets and bake 10-15 minutes before flipping beets over and baking for another 10-15 minutes until chips are crisp.

Crispy Golden Eggplant Fries Recipe

Serves: 4

Meet the ultimate snack food: Thick-cut veggie fries coated in a golden, crispy layer made of almond flour.

Tools

2 small bowls

2 shallow dishes

Chef's knife

Baking tray

Parchment paper

Ingredients

1 medium eggplant

1 egg, lightly beaten

¼ cup almond milk

1 ¼ cups almond flour

1 t garlic powder

1 t Italian seasoning

Salt and pepper, to taste

Extra virgin olive oil

Instructions

Preheat the oven to 400°F. Line a baking tray with parchment paper.

Cut the eggplant into 1-inch rounds, then slice those rounds into fry-size strips.

In a small bowl, whisk together the egg and almond milk. Set aside.

In a separate small bowl, stir together the almond flour, garlic powder, Italian seasoning, salt and pepper. Divide evenly onto two shallow dishes.

Roll the eggplant fries into the almond flour mixture on the first plate, then dip into the egg mixture, and then into the second plate of almond flour.

Place the eggplant fries evenly onto the prepared baking tray. Lightly drizzle them with extra virgin olive oil.

Bake for 20 minutes until they are crispy and golden brown. Remove from the oven and enjoy.

Cajun Oven-Baked Pickles

Serves: 10 pickles

These fried pickle spears are coated in almond flour and a robust blend of Cajun seasonings for a southern-style snack.

Tools

Baking sheet

Parchment paper

Paper towel

Shallow dish

Tongs

Ingredients

10 dill pickle spears

1 large egg

1/2 cup almond flour

1/2 t dried thyme

1/2 t dried oregano

1/4 t onion powder

1/4 t garlic powder

1/8 t smoked paprika

1/8 t cayenne pepper

Instructions

Preheat oven to 425°F and line a baking sheet with parchment paper. Blot pickle spears with a paper towel to remove excess liquid.

On a large plate, combine almond flour and seasonings. Beat egg in a separate shallow dish.

Dredge each pickle spear in egg, shake off any excess egg, and then coat in the almond flour-seasoning mixture.

Place pickles onto prepared baking sheet. Bake for 15 minutes. Use tongs to turn each spear and bake an additional 15 minutes. Serve immediately.

Easy Cauliflower Tater Tots

Serves: 4

Cauliflower replaces potatoes for a perfectly Paleo appetizer, snack, or side!

Ingredients

½ head large cauliflower, cut into florets

2 eggs, lightly beaten

¼ cup coconut flour

½ teaspoon garlic powder

¼ teaspoon onion powder

salt & pepper to taste

Instructions

Preheat oven to 400 degrees. Lightly grease a baking sheet with the coconut oil.

Steam the cauliflower florets in a large saucepan with an inch or so of water for 5 minutes until tender, but not mushy.

Place steamed cauliflower in a food processor and pulse a few times until the cauliflower is about the size of rice OR finely chop the florets until the size of rice.

In a medium bowl combine all ingredients and mix well.

Scoop out mixture 1 tablespoon at a time and shape into oval shapes. Place tots on the prepared baking sheet and bake for 20-22 minutes, flipping halfway through.

Guacamole Deviled Eggs

Serves: 8

These tasty bacon and avocado deviled eggs make for the perfect portable snack.

Ingredients

6 hardboiled eggs, cooled and peeled

1 t garlic, minced

1 t shallot, minced

1 large avocado, very ripe

1 t lemon juice

3 T bacon bits

pinch or two of salt

pinch or two of pepper

1/2 t paprika

Instructions

Slice your eggs in half lengthwise and spread them out onto a baking sheet.

Carefully extract the yolks from each egg and place them a large bowl.

Add the avocado, garlic, bacon bits, shallot, and lemon juice into the bowl. Mash and then stir until thoroughly combined.

Taste your mixture and season to taste.

Using a small ice cream scoop, melon baller or a spoon, scoop out the yolk and avocado mixture into the cavity of each piece of hardboiled egg.

Dust paprika over top of each, and enjoy!

Keto Breakfast Burrito with Bacon and Avocado

Serves: 2

Nutrition facts:9 grams of protein4 grams of carbohydrates14 grams of fat

Bacon, tomato, and avocado get rolled up in a protein-rich eggy patty for a gluten-free breakfast burrito.

Tools

Small mixing bowl

Medium Skillet

Spatula

Ingredients

4 pasture-raised eggs

2 T unsweetened almond milk

Ghee for greasing

4 strips cooked pasture-raised bacon, chopped

1 medium tomato, diced

Fresh greens of choice (spinach, cilantro, basil)

1/2 avocado, sliced

Instructions

Whisk together the eggs and almond milk in a mixing bowl.

Heat a skillet over medium heat and lightly grease with ghee.

Pour half of the mixture into the pan to coat the bottom thinly. Cover and cook for 3 minutes. Use a spatula to transfer to a plate.

Pour the remaining mixture into the skillet and cook for an additional 3 minutes, covered.

Top each egg "tortilla" with bacon, tomato, greens and avocado. Roll and enjoy!

Easy Baked Coconut-Crusted Salmon

Serves: 2

Tools

- Baking pan
- Cooking brush
- Mixing bowl

Ingredients

- 2 salmon fillets (around ½ pound each)
- 1 T melted coconut oil, divided, for greasing and brushing
- 1/2 cup unsweetened shredded coconut
- 2 T dried garlic-parsley mix

- Salt to taste

Instructions

- Preheat the oven to 350°F and grease the baking pan with coconut oil.

- Place salmon fillets skin-side-down on the prepared baking pan and brush the tops with coconut oil. Let the fillets cook for 5 minutes.

- As the fish bakes, combine the unsweetened shredded coconut, dried garlic-parsley mixture, and salt. Mix well until the ingredients are evenly distributed.

- Remove the salmon from the oven, brush the tops with more coconut oil, and press the shredded coconut mixture on top of the fillets with the back of a spoon.

- Drizzle coconut oil over the coconut crust and return the salmon to the oven for 15 more minutes, until the fillets are cooked through and the coconut crust is golden-brown.

- Serve the coconut-crusted salmon with fresh salad greens seasoned with salt and olive oil.

Low Carb Bacon-Fried Cabbage

Serves: 4

Nutrition facts:8 grams of protein12 grams of carbohydrates8 grams of fat

Fry up some cabbage with thick-cut bacon pieces for a low-carb dish that works as a side or as a main - either way, you're going to want more.

Tools

Large cast iron skillet

Ingredients

6 slices thick-cut bacon, cut into 1-inch pieces

1 cup diced onion

1 T minced garlic

6 cups thinly sliced cabbage

1 t salt

2 t ground black pepper

Instructions

In a cast iron skillet over medium heat, sauté the bacon pieces until the grease is rendered and bacon is cooked through and crispy, about 10 minutes. Remove the bacon pieces and set them aside on a paper towel-lined plate.

Reserve the bacon grease and add 2 tablespoons of it back to the skillet. Sauté the diced onions until soft and caramelized, about 5 minutes. Add the minced garlic and cook until the garlic is fragrant, about 1 minute. Set the cooked onions and garlic aside.

Add the remaining bacon grease to the skillet and stir in 2 cups of cabbage and cook until crispy, about 8 minutes. Use a wooden spoon to move the cabbage around occasionally to prevent burning. Set the cooked cabbage aside, and cook the rest of the cabbage in batches.

Once the cabbage is cooked, return the cabbage, onions, and garlic to the skillet. Sprinkle in the salt and pepper and mix well, before finally adding in the cooked bacon pieces. Serve immediately.

CONCLUSION

Proponents of the candida diet claim that it kills off candida overgrowth by eliminating sugar, gluten, alcohol and some dairy products. It focuses on organic, low-sugar, high-quality produce, meats and fats.

While the diet is healthy overall, many of its recommendations are not based on science. Nonetheless, if you have been diagnosed with a candida infection, it may be helpful to see if this diet works for you.

Printed in Great Britain
by Amazon

41400508R00081